ZIPPED TIED BOOTS

A Soldiers Treatment of PTSD
In Poplar Springs Hospital

GERALD PECKHAM

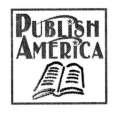

PublishAmerica
Baltimore

First printing

PublishAmerica has allowed this work to remain exactly as the author intended, verbatim, without editorial input.

Hardcover 978-1-4512-9600-6
Softcover 978-1-4489-6190-0
PAperback 978-1-4512-7116-4
PUBLISHED BY PUBLISHAMERICA, LLLP
www.publishamerica.com
Baltimore

Printed in the United States of America

Special Thanks

To Poplar Springs Behavioral Healthcare Center Staff, RN's, Psychologists', Health Care Specialists in the Military Unit. Helping Soldiers, who are recovering from Alcohol addiction, PTSD, Co Dependency, Stress, and Marriage Counseling.

My wife, Gina and my children, Andrew and Ryan.

Mr. & Mrs. Ralph Peckham, and Melissa (Madden) Kelly.

CONTENTS

Introduction

Gerald Peckham was born and raised in Muncie, Indiana; On September 6, 1982, he joined the US Army, as an Infantryman, after serving eighteen years he reclassified into the Mortuary Affairs field, where he served two tours in Iraq. Gerald Peckham began writing the manuscript for his first book, three months later after the loss of his Grandmother on October 6, 1995.

Her entire life was centered on Jesus Christ. Her faith, love and inspiration she left went unnoticed as she traded her crown for a mansion to be with Jesus. In my first book "THE HEART OF A SHEPHERD" describes the spiritual blessing, when the Holy Spirit shared a very touching and remarkable vision, while he stood by her bedside. His Grandmother was diagnosed with Alzheimer's disease.

Gerald Peckham shares his spiritual gift to others through his writing, and has dedicated his gift towards writing non-fiction, and Children's Books.

In 2005, during his first tour in Iraq, when a Fallen Soldier, who served as a Combat Medic, left behind eight children, inspired him to write his first Children's Book "Tommy Tuttle and the Fire Station", In 2009, four years later, he found an illustrator for the Children's Book, which will be released in the fall 2010. The Book dedicated to the Firemen and Women, who risk their lives daily and those Men and Women of the Armed Forces.

Preface

It was February 1, 2005, the wives, children, family and friends are giving their last hugs and kisses to their Soldiers assigned to 125th FSB Headquarters and Headquarters Company, 3rd Brigade 1st Armored Division, Fort Riley, Kansas. The Soldiers just returned in April 2004, from a twelve month tour in Iraq, and much of the Brigades equipment didn't return till late June 2004.

While they were in Iraq, I had just PCS'D (Permanent Change of Station), from the Headquarters Company, 1st Battalion 27th Infantry (Wolfhounds), 25th Infantry Division (Light), Schofield Barracks Hawaii. I was a forty year old 11 Bravo Infantryman, that had spent eighteen years of my life doing the hardest job that requires a tremendous amount of discipline, being physically fit, and leadership. In this MOS (Military Occupational Skill), there is no room for error, especially in a combat zone. I came to the realization that it was time for me to move to another military occupation skill, now that the orthopedic doctors examined my feet after failing to complete two EIB (Expert Infantryman's Badge) 12 mile road marches, which must be completed in three hours, wearing your uniform with boots, and a 35 pound rucksack on your back. Over eighteen years, you're liable to have some limitations, like fallen arches in your feet only to become flat footed. I was referred to see an orthopedics doctor at Tripler Army Medical Center, Hawaii, which I was recommended to the MMRB (Military Medical Review Board), to determine if I was physically fit to remain on active duty or referred to the MEB (Medical Evaluation Board).

MEB is a board that medically retires and discharges Soldiers from active duty with compensation of a disability percentage which is based off their current base pay.

It took eight months to see the MMRB, so my career was in their hands. In April 2004, I was in Fort Lee, Virginia, attending the Mortuary Affairs Center, learning a new MOS. After completing the seven weeks of training, and assigned to Fort Riley, Kansas.

Chapter One
"Never leave a Fallen Comrade"

The chartered flight landed at Kuwait International Airport about 0230hrs on February 2, which the flight is roughly 19-20hrs flying time. The baggage detail of twenty junior enlisted Soldiers, from Private to Specialist (E-4), and three noncommissioned Officers (E-5, E-6's), to remove over six hundred duffle bags, and some heavy foot lockers holding some sensitive items. As the detail was unloading the rest of the Soldiers on the plane were exiting the plane and to the Kuwaiti buses that were waiting for our arrival. The Kuwaiti buses are very different than the buses in the United States. The seats are smaller and each bus holds about thirty people but wearing our IBA's (Interceptor Body Armor), with individual weapons, it gets tight.

The drive to our next location would take 2-3 hours, with a Kuwaiti Police escorting the buses to the main road where the unit would stay for the next 2-3 weeks, before heading north into Iraq. One by one, the bus driver's Identifications were checked and an accurate count of Soldiers on each bus given to the guards at the entry control point.

The exact location of where we were staying can't be given, due to Operation Security measures, and to protecting those who are still serving in Iraq.

The temperature in Kuwait was in the mid 50's during the nights, and the days reached the upper 90's. It felt cold during the night because your body absorbs all the heat and no trees for shade.

February 16, 2005, today the units are pushing forward to the north into Iraq. A convoy of military vehicles of all different types lined up and ready to roll. There were some last minute changes to the travel plans for those Soldiers riding shot gun to provide security just in case we have to fire our weapon. My 1SG told me that I was taken off the list to fly on the Air Force's C-130, leaving from Kuwait International Airport to BIAP (Baghdad International Airport), and that I will be pulling security for the driver in a bobtail, which is a rig that can pull a trailer, but we wouldn't be hauling one. At this point I was very concerned and nervous for the fact that this is my first deployment to Iraq. I knew that if I called my wife she would be terrified about me riding three days on roads where there could potentially be roadside bombs, known as IED's (Improvised Explosive Devices). The threat was very possible, but I also know that sharing information over the phone is a violation of Operation Security, and could be putting my unit in danger, because the enemy can use the internet, and phones to gather Intel about our missions in Iraq. We reached our base camp in three days of traveling on sandy roads, where I had seen Iraqi children running up to our convoy, when we stopped to let another convoy pass that was going south towards Kuwait. Most of the children were about nine or ten years old walking around barefooted with cartons of Iraqi cigarettes, trying to sell them to the Soldiers. As I was watching the children there was one child that was walking through an open field with barbed wire. It hit me hard thinking of my own children and how blessed they are to have the comforts of living in the United States of America.

By late February, the casualty collection point that supported about 13,000 Soldiers on the camp, received its first KIA (Killed in Action), case from 1st CAV from Fort Hood, where a Soldier was hit by an IED, while on a foot patrol. The unit was on its last mission, which they were conducting with the new incoming unit that would assume the missions for the next 12 months. The Captain brought in a small box of the Soldiers remains that could be recovered at this time. In March, the CCP (Casualty Collection Point) received more cases of US Soldiers and Iraqi National Guard Soldiers which later would be known as Iraqi Security Forces. Most of the remains we cared for where the result of IED's and Sniper fire from the insurgents. In late March I decided to take the EML (Environmental Leave), which now it's called R and R months. I had only been in Iraq only a month and I felt like I needed to find a secure place and away from the reality of war. When I arrived home I noticed that I lost the desire for the things I used to enjoy, like playing video games and watching television with my sons, Ryan and Andrew.

I was finding myself waking up in the middle of the night, reliving the traumatic events which I experienced I Iraq, processing the remains of US Soldiers and seeing their faces, once again. I was even looking for my weapon, which seemed to me that it became an attachment of me, since all Soldiers in Iraq carry a weapon with them at all times. I would find myself being more observant of my surroundings, like people and that you never know who could be the enemy, which is the result of the pre-deployment training that I received before deploying to Iraq. I tried to enjoy the time with my wife and children, but it wasn't the same anymore, because I wasn't the same either.

The fifteen days of leave seemed like it flew by overnight, but in Iraq it's just the opposite, each day that goes by seems like a lifetime. I couldn't stop thinking about the job I had left and what was waiting for me when I get back to doing what is considered the most difficult job in the entire Army.

The moment our plane left Dallas Fort Worth Airport in Texas, the Soldiers slept most of the entire flight until landing at Kuwait International Airport; my mind was back into the awareness mode. It took about three days to get back to the FOB (Forward Operating Base), which I had to fly in a CH-47 (Chinook), and a UH-60 (Blackhawk) to get back to the unit.

We were now in the first month of May, as the hot weather reached the upper nineties and some days it reached the one hundred degree mark. The hot wind blowing in your face felt like opening clothes dryer, which my uniform would absorb all the heat. The entire month of May was the best month, I had worked without any incidents, but we still had till January 2006, before we redeploy back to Fort Riley, Kansas.

The biggest problem that I had to deal with for the remaining tour was keeping positive and taking my online College classes, which I signed up for prior to deploying. I was studying for my associate's degree in business at Central Texas College, which was possible through the Army's Earmyu program for Soldiers who can earn their degree while they serve. I only had one class in American History, which covered the Civil War; I never did do well in High School. I worked in the 125th FSB (Forward Support Battalion), which supported the 3rd BCT, 1st Armored Division, providing fuel, parts, water supply, and transportation, which is how the mission gets accomplished through the Quartermaster Corps. I was given the responsibilities of leadership jobs which turned out to be an everyday duty. I held the positions as the Brigade Mortuary Affairs NCO, Brigade Transportation NCO, and the 125th Battalion UPL (Unit Prevention Leader), who is qualified to do drug screening tests;

and standing in one of the worst smelling guard towers on the FOB, which was tower nineteen.

I was overloaded with too many duties that it caused me to have sleep problems, stress, and anxiety.

June 2005, another month marked off the calendar, and the CCP has received at least five remains of US Soldiers, and three Iraqi Security Forces Soldiers. We were equipped with a refrigeration room that was always set between 34-38 degrees to keep the remains from decomposition, and two processing rooms where we would inventory the Soldiers PE (Personal Effects), like money, watch, sentimental items, i.e., religious cross, ID bracelet from a wife, husband, or mother.

Once the remains of US Soldiers were processed for evacuation, 125th FSB would support the CCP by loading the US remains in a five ton truck with overhead cover; the remains wouldn't be seen going to the flight line, which is a five to ten minute drive across the FOB, where the Blackhawks would be waiting for our arrival. Someone needed to go with these US Soldiers to ensure they were handled with respect, dignity, and honor. I was a Sergeant, but the highest ranking noncommissioned officer working in the CCP, so I volunteered myself to go on the mission, rather than selecting the lowest ranking Soldier. As we approached the gate there were two US Soldier giving us the hand signal to enter. On the landing pad I saw two Blackhawks with the rotors rotating very rapidly and two door gunners from each, standing there waiting patiently for the US Fallen Comrades. We loaded two Soldiers on the first Blackhawk, and then the other three on the second. As each Soldier was loaded, the door gunner would stand and hold a salute as one of our own were given the proper respect, dignity, and honor, which everyone of them deserve. I was strapped in the middle seat which fits only three people, and we lifted off the ground with the nose of the Blackhawk downward, and the rear stabilizer upward. I looked down at my feet, took a moment to pray for these Soldiers family, and how their lives will be changing soon, once the next of kin is officially notified.

The two weeks after escorting the two US Soldiers, it was back to my other duties which would be handled while taking care of our Fallen Comrades at the CCP twenty four hours a day, and seven days a week.

I celebrated 4th of July 2005, by eating the usual hot dogs and hamburgers that the dining facility cooked outside for all the Soldiers, which there were over ten thousand on the FOB. I tried to call my wife back home in Manhattan, Kansas, but with the amount of Soldiers in Iraq, which was over two hundred thousand during this time, you might as well send a card in the mail. The things that I know I have missed the most and other Soldiers that I have talked to is the birthdays of your wife and children. The anniversaries, a Soldier missing his wife giving birth to their first child, or being there on Christmas morning to hear your children's excitement in their voices when they see that Santa Claus left presents under the Christmas Tree. Each day I would think about those times I spent with my family, knowing that I have given my wife and children a better quality of health care, housing, and financial security.

It was about the middle of July 2005, when the CCP, had received seven (ISF), Iraqi Security Forces Soldiers, that were killed at a check point, as there was a funeral precession approached them, but it turned out to be an ambush. All Soldiers suffered one bullet wound to the head. We kept them overnight in the refrigeration room until the next morning. The next morning the ISF Commander and other Soldiers loaded the remains in an Iraqi Ambulance to transport them to a Baghdad Hospital, where the family can identify the body.

I left the CCP about 10:30AM, after cleaning the refrigeration room and sweeping the light sand off the concrete walkway just outside the office, and then I drove to my room to get some sleep. The CCP, had a policy that if there were ever human remains in the refrigeration room, then someone will sleep in the office to guard the Soldiers remains, which trying to sleep in the office when you know what's on the other side of the wall, which is something I did often. The hardest part is when it's dark outside with no lighting on the outside, you're inside an office, and the littlest sound makes you jump right out of your skin. When I heard these sounds, I unlocked the door and looked outside to see nothing, I checked inside the refrigeration room as I turned on the light to check on the remains we were holding, and I found myself doing this many times during the twelve month tour. Later that same day about 2:00PM, when I was awakened by someone was knocking at my door; it was one of the Soldiers from HQ's 125th FSB, sent by the First Sergeant to deliver the message. The Soldier had informed that a Soldier from 125th FSB was reported as KIA (Killed in Action), which that information is not given out until it's confirmed by his or her military identification card or tags. After spending all night at the CCP, unable to sleep, feeling physically and mentally tired. I ran to my military vehicle parked on the other side of the barriers, which gives the US Soldiers some protection from shrapnel in case of a mortar attacks. One my way to the CCP, I stopped at HQ's 125th FSB to get an update on the status of the Soldier, and the arrival time, so that I can prepare the proper forms that are required. As I was walking to the door, our Battalion Executive Officer, Major Poole, wanted to have a meeting in the Battalion Conference Room, with our First Sergeant, Mortuary Affairs, Company Commander and the Summary Court Martial Officer, who was selected just after hearing the news. He told me that Specialist Jared Hartley, who was a Light Wheeled Vehicle Mechanic, who was killed by a VBIED (Vehicle Bourne Improvised Explosive Device), when the vehicle detonated as it approached their convoy. In the conference room, the acting Battalion Commander, asked me what the procedures were in taking care of the Soldiers personal effects. The remains were evacuated to the Military Surgical Hospital, north of Baghdad; later the remains will be transported to the MACP (Mortuary Affairs Collection Point), for processing and within twelve hours to Dover, Delaware. The loss of a Soldier affects everyone in the respective unit and the entire military, and those loved ones back home. The sacrifice of a Soldiers life during combat is a hard price to pay, and the outcome is that it changes many lives forever.

In August 2005, one month closer to going home but we still have five more months ahead. The temperatures in Iraq reached the one hundred and thirty degree mark which is mostly a dry heat. The CCP has received six remains, which was the average during this deployment. Most of the Soldiers of the 125th FSB, had taken their fourteen days of leave back home to see their loved ones, and looking forward to returning home soon. I on the other hand had a different perspective, which I was thinking about all those US fallen comrades who died on the dusty battlefields of Iraq.

It's September 2005, which is the anniversary when the 9/11, terrorists attacked the Worlds Trade Building. The war in Iraq reaches the second year since the first invasion began in March 2003.

I was referred by the 125th FSB, Company Commander, to see a mental health clinic; located across from the trailers were living.

The mind had absorbed so many traumas, having to deal with these fallen Soldiers deaths, not to mention the responsibility and having some hallucinations experience. The mental health clinic referred me to a Combat Stress Clinic, located at another FOB, which was about a ten to twenty minute flight north in a Chinook. I arrived at the PAX terminal, which most Soldiers who have flown from FOB to FOB, have waited for hours or days to get a flight out to their destination. I called the Combat Stress Clinic from the phone located in the terminal and within ten minutes the driver was parked in front of the PAX terminal. The clinic was located down the street from the PX (Post Exchange), where Soldiers can buy everything from cigarettes to espresso machines. I looked at this white wooded structure with the sign hanging above saying, "COMBAT STRESS CLINIC," the first thing that came to my mind was, everyone will notice that I am seeking help and I'm a weak leader, especially when your command views you as a outstanding noncommissioned officer. It was about 10:00PM, when I walked in through the front door thinking I would be strapped in a strait jacket with the staff wearing white uniforms, but that wasn't the case. I turned in my M16, which is my weapon along with the seven magazines fully loaded with 5.56mm, ammunition, which was required for Soldiers to carry when traveling anywhere in Iraq. They led me into a room to search my bag to remove all sharp objects that could be used if I wanted to harm myself, also to protect the other patients, who were already asleep in the backroom. I felt like I was this was the end to my career, and going home with the memories of battle on your mind, with difficulty coping with life after the war, like our Vietnam Veterans did when they returned home. I went to the backroom where the others were sleeping to find a bunk to sleep. The lights were off so I didn't want to wake the others but a few Soldiers welcomed me to the clinic, which we talked as I sat on my bunk, exchanging our stories of how each of us ended up in the combat stress clinic. The first Soldier told me about that he was out on a mission, when their convoy was hit by a roadside bomb. The second Soldier said that he had trouble sleeping because of mission after mission, without anytime to recover, which was the breaking point. I didn't need to say much when I mentioned, mortuary affairs. Without any hesitation both Soldiers agreed, I needed to be here. Over the next three days I participated in group sessions, anger management, and relaxation exercises for the Soldiers with trouble sleeping.

I met with the mental health specialist asked me if I ever considered committing suicide, and if there were a family history of mental health issues within the family, which we didn't. The Battle Stress Clinic released me back to my unit, with limited duties that would be less stressful for the remaining tour.

The first sergeant of Headquarters and Headquarters Company, 125th FSB, was sitting at his desk, when I handed him the profile, and took a few minutes to review, then he asked me if I was feeling better. I told him that I was rested and that it did me a lot of good, which I will never regret for getting help. I stuck to the light duty, helping with the support operations office, and leaving work earlier, which relived most of the stress that I had prior to the Combat Stress Clinic.

October 2005, the Soldiers in the 125thFSB, were already talking about home, and planning their first day, which most of them were going to get a beer, and eating American fast food. I had a different plan in mind, which were to meet with those spouses from the 3rd Brigade, 1st Armored Division, who lost their husbands during this twelve month tour. The faces of those fallen comrades, was like seeing a reflection of myself, and that part of me died, knowing that we wear the same uniform. Thinking of going home to my wife, since April 2005, hugging my children and finding my place in the family again as a father, after being gone for twelve months. These Soldiers may have gone home with Honor, but their spirits will forever be left on the battlefields of Iraq, which it seems like we will be going home without them.

The most horrific experience that I will never forget is when two U.S Soldiers who were Military Police, who were coming back from a checkpoint, just north of our FOB, as they were driving their M1114 (Gun Truck,), making the vehicle weigh two tons, were engaged with an EFP (Explosively Formed Penetrator.) The Iraqi Fire Department came to the rescue, which received training from U.S. Fire Fighters, were unable to reach the Soldiers due to the intense heat and flames and the large amount of live ammunition that was going off inside the vehicle. Once the threat of being wounded, from the hot bursting live ammunition, the fire fighters quickly extinguished the flames. Our CCP, didn't receive the remains, but rather evacuated to a military medical hospital, about a twenty five minute flight south in a Blackhawk. A First Lieutenant came to the 125th FSB, Support Operations Office, asking for the Mortuary Affairs noncommissioned Officer in charge for the 3rd Brigade, 1st Armored, and that he needed to have the M1114, searched and recover all human portions remaining inside. I drove to the battle damage yard to see the vehicle loaded on a flat bed trailer, completely charred, even the tires were burned, down to the rims. I grabbed a handful of zip lock plastic bags, which are used in recovering small portions of human remains that belong to the deceased Soldiers. On the floor of the driver's side, next to the accelerator and the brake were human bones from the feet of the driver. I put on two sets of latex examination gloves for health and safety measures. I used a pen to sift through the ashes, only to stir up a strong odor of burnt flesh. Each bag was labeled on the outside with the date of recovery, where in the vehicle it was recovered. On the same side behind the driver's seat is where the passenger would sit was three teeth still intact with the maxillary, which had come from the upper part of the jaw. I searched the other side of the vehicle but found nothing.

That evening I was sitting in my room with the strong scent of death in my nose, with the flashbacks of the bones in my mind.

November 2005, the Soldiers are celebrating Thanksgiving Day, which seems to lose its meaning when you're away from family, and friends. Outside the dining hall there were Soldiers waiting in lines for forty five minute to enjoy their Thanksgiving meal, with their comrades. The menu covered the turkey, which it was far from the traditional butterball that I normally would carve, cornbread dressing, and assorted vegetables, salad bar, ice cream, and pumpkin pie, which all the Soldiers enjoyed, some going back for seconds.

The Holiday seasons is the most difficult time of the year when deployed Soldiers experience times of depression, anxiety, feeling restless, because they have been cooped up from six to fifteen months, where their freedom is within a small compound, among tens of thousands of men and women in the United States Armed Forces. It's those who have served in uniform understand the sacrifices they're making especially those with multiple tours in Iraq or Afghanistan.

The next month would be the hardest of all Holiday's, Christmas. My presents from my wife, kids, mom and dad, were received in October 2005, so that it doesn't get caught up with those last minute packages being mailed to Iraq or Afghanistan for their loved ones.

When you think that you're having a bad day, there is someone else out there who comes along who proves us wrong. It was December 20, 2005, about 10:00AM, when the TOC (Tactical Operations Center), received a message over the radio from a convoy from 2nd Battalion 70th Armor, that one of their M1114's had been hit by an IED, and they have three KIA's. I was sitting in the SPO (Support Operations Office), as soon as I heard the incoming call; I quickly grabbed a Motorola radio, headed to the CCP, which were a few minutes down the road. Within a few minutes at the CCP, the TOC reported that there were four KIA's. I prepared the room and the paperwork for the four Soldiers, and now the long wait begins.

The three M1114's stopped in front of the CCP, as the Soldiers jumped out of their vehicles and asking me for guidance since I was the subject matter expert, so at this point I directed them to bring two of the Soldiers inside the processing room which has an American Flag hanging on the wall. Four Soldiers carried the litter with their fallen comrade inside as they rested it across two stands which hold the remains, before beginning the paperwork. The other two Soldiers were placed inside the refrigeration room to keep them from decomposing. After I was talking with the Soldiers who carried him inside, told me that this Soldier was a Combat Medic, and that he was the forth KIA, also he has eight children. The most disturbing news that stuck in my mind that this Soldier had three children of his own form his first marriage, and that his current wife, which had three from her previous marriage, and they had two children together. The Combat Medic's injuries were so severe that he couldn't even perform his job when the IED hit they're convoy. The Soldiers from the other vehicle's acted quickly by applying the CAT (Combat Application Tourniquet), to both legs above the knee, and both arms just above the elbows. Probably the last thing on his mind was his wife and children, because he knew that he was bleeding profusely through his extremities, a medic with three tours in Iraq. This is where Soldiers would want to die, knowing they fought along with trained professional, Soldiers, and they died for a cause, not by crime but something they believed in with all their heart.

The twelve month tour ended in January with the 3rd BCT, 1st Armored Division, Fort Riley, Kansas, ended with a Soldier committing suicide from who was from the 4th Infantry Division, Fort Hood, Texas. This Soldier had only been here just ten days!

Chapter Two

"Soldiers Coming Home"

The chartered flight bringing home over three hundred exhausted of our Heroes, which were mostly from the 125th FSB, 3rd Brigade, 1st Armored Division, of Fort Riley, Kansas, landed at Forbes Field in Topeka, Kansas, on January 21, 2006. The flight took almost nineteen hours, from Kuwait, including a stop in Shannon Ireland to refuel. The Soldiers were gathered at every window wanting to see US soil, rather than the Iraqi sand, which some had commented that this is what they missed, which is something that most haven't seen in almost six to twelve months. As the plane made its final approach for landing there was total silence in the entire plane that you could hear a pin drop. The plane's rear wheel barely touches home, as the Soldiers cheered and clapped their hands. The voice of the pilot came over the intercom, and gave us all a Welcome Home, and for our serving our Country.

Even though the Soldiers were home, we still had fallen comrades, that couldn't share this moment. They will not be here to see their spouses, children, moms and dads. I had taken this moment to remember the Soldiers, who died during this conflict in Iraq; the burden on my heart was so strong that I needed to share my experience with someone who would understand the loss of a Solider, fighting for their country.

There were buses waiting at the terminal door as each Soldier loaded the buses that would take them to Army Airfield on Fort

Riley. We headed on Interstate 70 West; the Soldiers received a welcome home from Veterans and active duty, riding their Harley Davidson motorcycles, with American Flags mounted. Upon arrival the Soldiers were dropped off at a hanger to turn in our weapons, and get some lunch before reuniting with our loved ones, which was two hangers down, and filled with parents, spouses who had given birth while their Soldiers were deployed. The thirty minutes of waiting inside the hanger, added more anticipation when we first landed. The command of "Fall In," was given within a few minutes the Soldiers with Honor, and Respect, will be welcomed home from Families and the local community.

We marched inside the hanger one by one, which were heavily decorated with American Flags, large and small; some had painted the Flag on their faces. The applause came from the crowd, went on till the last Soldier entered the hanger, then the Commanding General introduced to the families, "These are your Soldiers." The crowd cheered with smile on their faces, and with tears of joy. The Commanding General's words were brief, and his final command was, "Wives find your Soldier." At an instant there was a stampede from the bleachers, and within seconds, wives found their Soldiers, but I had to walk around the large crowd to find my wife. I thought I would never find her, but I did after ten minutes, giving her the biggest hug, which makes every Soldier coming home, an unforgettable moment reunited with your family who have supported you through the war.

My wife and I were paying rent for a three bedroom house with a one car garage attached, before leaving Iraq in February 2005. She decided to move since the house didn't have central air; kitchen had the old metal cabinets, plus the carpet needed replaced. I came home to a three story four bedroom townhouse. I couldn't miss our new home, especially when I saw a banner hanging on a garage door saying, "Welcome Home Sergeant Peckham." I was looking forward to being home without carrying my weapon with me everywhere I go. The first night home I could still see the faces of most of the Soldiers, who were processed at the CCP, in Iraq. The next morning, just before I opened my eyes thinking that this is still Iraq. It's like the time when I was at Fort Benning, Georgia, for Infantry Basic Training; I dreamed that I was still at home sleeping in my own bedroom, when I was awakened by the lights from the Drill Sergeant. In this case, I wasn't dreaming that I am home in the safest place in the world, with my family.

In the first week, I was suffering from insomnia, anxiety, and some depression, which I thought would be normal after returning from a combat zone, eventually it pass after a few weeks. There were days that I felt like I was not motivated to do the things I enjoyed doing, before I went to Iraq. I always loved to play video games with my children, watch television, cook, and sometimes even clean the house. A father always gives their children small chores like taking out the trash to earn their weekly allowance, but here I was thinking that maybe this is something I could do, so I could feel like I can start being part of this family once again. My wife managed to handle the finances while I was deployed, which is important for the spouses to know how to manage the income while their husband's are away. I had mixed emotions that I could feel inside and some of those feelings I expressed with tears, and guilt. I know the Soldiers who died in Iraq chose their careers for themselves, but the responsibility that I had during that time, brought a heavy burden on my heart. The difficult times where when I used my command voice at my son, which at this time he was twelve to clean his room, or simple chores around the house. Afterwards,

I knew that I was wrong for making a big ass of myself for yelling at him, when he did nothing wrong. I was beginning to wonder who the hell I was anymore, and how long can anyone put up with me.

The mandatory reintegration classes for all Soldiers, those Soldiers who were married were encouraged to attend with their wives, and programs that offer marriage counseling, depression, anxiety, alcohol and drug addiction, and PTSD. In 1990-1991, during the Gulf War, there were Soldiers, who returned with symptoms of depression, stress, anxiety, and some have attempted suicide, also reported cases during the conflict from the exposure to stressful situations, and Soldiers being exposed to the black smoke, coming from the Kuwait oil fields. I didn't check with a Community Mental Health Specialists, which my thought was this is going to pass with the support from my wife and children I'll be fine.

Two weeks later the classes were completed as a Soldier would say, it's checking the block training. The entire 3rd BCT, 1st Armored Division, were taking their thirty days of block leave, a phase two after the redeployment, but I only taken ten days as some were going on cruises to the Bahamas, and hunting. Some others were getting back to reality which for some that was hitting the bars in Aggieville, which is the social life for the students at Kansas State University, Manhattan, Kansas.

My Mom and Dad calls me from their cell phone, during the second day of my leave, they were coming to see me, and of course I asked when, my mother never could keep the suspense of surprises, she told me that they were one hour away from St. Louis, Missouri, and would be arriving around 6:00PM, the next day. My wife scrambled to clean the bathrooms, as I started to dust the furniture, and vacuum the floors. The kids bedrooms needed cleaned, as my wife, Gina, worked up a sweat scrubbing the bathtub.

Mom and Dad arrived about 7:00PM, the following day for their surprise visit. I was still having a difficult time sleeping through the night, waking up at 1:00AM, lying back down to be awake once again at 2:30AM, then at 4:00AM. I didn't attempt to return to bed so I went downstairs to watch television, until the kids woke up or Gina. I would make a pot of coffee and sit in the lounge chair, only to think about the Soldiers who died in Iraq. It has affected my life as a Soldier and as a person who had given two hundred percent during those twelve months in Iraq. I packed two black tote boxes with personal gear and military clothing that wouldn't fit inside the duffle bag, since there was limited space under the plane. I stored them in the laundry room downstairs so that I could have them later for the next deployment. The ideal of unpacking them would have brought back memories that I just didn't wanted to face. I didn't want to discuss the horrific details about the Soldiers to my Mom or Dad because I believe that they wouldn't understand the reality of war, compared to seeing it from the news. I kept the emotions deep inside of my conscience and tried to act like a normal man.

My Mom and Dad left after a three day visit, so this allowed me to have some free time to relax, and to find the right time to talk with Gina about my experience in Iraq. The next day which was a Saturday, we had cooked out on out little grill, and my kids were playing video games on their XBOX, which Gina and I walked outside to sit on the front porch to enjoy the outdoors. I told her about the Soldier who was the Combat Medic, with eight children, who was killed by an IED. The other incident was the recovery of those two MP's, where I had to search inside the vehicle where I recovered portions of their bones, and three teeth still intact with the maxillary, the upper portion of the human teeth. I didn't get much of a response from my wife, only for her to reply that this is something that she couldn't bear to imagine if I were to die in Iraq knowing that most of the Soldiers who come home to be buried are non viewable. The most important thing to her was to have a viewing with an open casket, with the U.S. Flag draped, just like Lawrence Edward Gunderman, her father a drafted Soldier in 1951, who served in the Arkansas National Guard. In 2002, he died from congestive heart failure, while going under treatment in the hospital, later his casket was draped with the U.S. Flag, a true honor.

I've never given this a thought until lately that if I should perish during combat then her having to deal with the loss of a husband, and to leave two teenage children fatherless, and the burial of Lawrence Edward Gunderman, who was a father and a Soldier.

Chapter Three
"I Will Never Quit"

In March 2006, 3rd BCT, 1st Armored Division, Fort Riley, Kansas, became another active duty unit in military history that deployed to Kuwait in 2003, during the invasion, only to move northward, crossing the Iraq border. Those were the memories that the Commanding General mentioned during his speech to the Soldiers of the "Bulldog" Brigade, standing with their comrades who fought against the enemy. The Brigade was demobilized, this very day, since the Army's restructure program.

I had received orders to Fort Stewart, Georgia, but with the new Combat Aviation Brigade coming mostly from Germany, and Fort Rucker, I would be reassigned to the unit as the mortuary affairs NCOIC, (noncommissioned officer in charge), training Soldiers and Officers before the unit deploys for their fifteen month tour to Iraq. In August 2006, the 601st ASB, (Aviation Support Battalion), with less than forty percent strength of Soldiers, as more were coming from other military posts, to fill the ranks. It was six months ago that I returned home after a twelve month deployment and now preparing for a second tour.

Once a Soldier experiences his or her first combat tour, whether in Iraq or Afghanistan, within a few weeks of returning to their duty station, Soldiers would rather go back to continue their mission. The feelings were mutual since the first time in combat working in the most stressful, hardest job in the Army, mortuary affairs. I met with the 601st ASB, Command Sergeant Major in his office; he reviewed my ERB, (Enlisted Records Brief), looking for those who have been deployed previously and military schools needed for promotions. The CSM, told me that the Combat Aviation Brigade, has never been assigned a mortuary affairs personnel, and that I would be the first. My experiences come with the knowledge, self confidence, and the utmost professionalism, for that fallen comrade, especially in combat. The Army mission never stops as a Soldier, which I started preparing the SOP, (Standard Operating Procedures), guidelines that will cover the mortuary affairs operations for the 601st ASB, 1st Infantry Division, during Iraq.

In September 2009, after training less than a year in convoy operations and preparing equipment for the deployment, the 601st ASB, 1st Infantry, were given a formal ceremony with spouses, children and family present wishing all the Soldiers to return home soon. As I was slowly marching through the hanger doors, I could see my wife's face with tears running down her cheeks and my children who for the first time were seeing their father going off to war for his second tour to Iraq. The 601st ASB had many new Soldiers that were deploying for the first time, saying good bye to their wives or fiancée. I understand what they're going through and within the first weeks of the deployment is how to keep your mind off your husband, wondering how he is doing from day to day.

The Soldiers of the 601stb ASB flew out of Forbes Field, Topeka Kansas, after flying for nearly seven to eight hours the chartered flight made a stop in Shannon, Ireland to refuel. Almost every Soldier who deployed to Iraq is very familiar with the short visit to Shannon Ireland Airport, as this gives Soldiers the opportunity to have a smoke break outside the airport, and try some real Irish espresso, especially when it's the first place we stop that serves alcohol, but it's off limits. Our flight time into Kuwait International Airport, would take about eight to nine hours. As soon as I could see the tan colored sand, you're saying to yourself, I am back again. The routine for Soldiers when arriving to Iraq, via Kuwait hasn't changed much when it comes to the first two or three weeks in the Country.

What made this fifteen month tour different in many ways, comparison to that of my first twelve month tour that I had mentioned earlier in chapter one. The similarities of both were, the places we remained for the first two weeks were the same, as in 2005-2006 tour, and those responsibilities were to train and ensure that the remains of those fallen comrades during this tour would be handled with respect and with honor.

What were those things that I encountered during my second tour, making this an incredible tour? It was in February 2008; I was working the 12:00 pm to 10:00pm at the Support Operations Office, the 601st ASB Soldiers made through the holidays and now well into our sixth month inside Iraq. I walked into my office and sat at my desk checking my emails before I went to lunch. As was sitting in my chair, I felt the presence of the Holy Spirit as I was sitting inside my office. I closed my eyes and the instant I had closed them, the Holy Spirit revealed this vision for me to see. In this vision, I am inside a church, sitting in one of the pews on the right side. The inside of the church was dark, but the light coming from those burning candles that were sitting on a table which was placed to the front so each person who comes to the church for prayer will light a candle. As I am looking over to the left side of the church, I see a woman, who is praying, and she is crying out to Jesus for help. I can feel her heavy burden that she is carrying, and her prayer is for someone who is close to death. As she weeps for an answer from God, I heard this very calm and pleasant voice saying, "Be Still My Child," and the woman stopped crying, but those words were just the beginning to what the Holy Spirit revealed to me later that day, which was a message to her but to share with others. The Poem reads:

"Be Still My Child"

Be still my child for I have been here since the beginning and will till the end, I brought the Israelites out of bondage, across the Red Sea and to the Promised Land I promised thee. They were like you in many ways; only troubled by sin and in disarray. I feel your pain for my Son Jesus Christ had suffered the same. Your faith brings you peace and your heart holiness. Be still my child for I am here to help you this very day, like my Son Jesus Christ was sacrificed to save. I see the tears of the elderly when they are sick, and even the young ones that have died I our wars, and those babies that have been killed despite not being born. It brings tears to my eyes and pain to see my children suffer when I have been here since they were delivered; my words to you my child continue on your life's journey and pray without ceasing, so that my Son Jesus Christ was not sacrificed for nothing. The skies will open when no one will know the time. It could be during a snowstorm or even during the night. Jesus will come only for the holy ones and those who have remained strong, and US Soldiers who have died in our past wars. My word says that life is like a vapor, here today and gone tomorrow, but don't be discouraged for life in heaven will be better than you could have expected. Your riches are stored in heaven for all that have paid, but my lesson to you my children is that I command you to obey. Be still my child, for I have a place for you in heaven that has been here for more than a day, but it will still be here when you see me on the Judgment Day!

Written by SSG Gerald Peckham, War Poetry, this was Copyright in 2008.

In May 2008, I published my first book "THE HEART OF A SHEPHERD," a book I started in January 1995, after my Grandmother passed away. It's the story of special moments that changed my life, and memories of her life as a devoted Christian, filled with faith, love and life.

I had many days over the thirteen years, filled with uncertainty, lack of faith, not knowing if the book would become a reality or just flop. The first thing that I knew for sure was the spiritual vision that came through the Holy Spirit, as I stood by her bedside, shortly after her death. What did I have to lose by trusting in the Lord, absolutely nothing, but all to gain, through Him, allowing me to see a wonderful miracle right before my eyes?

The difference in my second deployment was that I spent more time in prayer, reading God's Word, and listening to the Lord with an open heart, and without the heavy burden of the fallen Soldiers, like the first time. The Lord gives rest for the tired and weary so, this was a blessing, which I would enjoy.

In June 2008, I written my second book "The Power of Prayer," after publishing the first book, I did some extensive research reading through the New Testament and the Old Testament of the King James Version Bible.

In July 2008, it's the month of fireworks, cookouts, and our freedom and Independence. I had volunteered to be the Editor of the newsletter for my unit, Headquarters and Headquarters Company 601st ASB, which was sent through spouse's emails to give them the chance to see their deployed Solider. The unit had planned to do a cookout and a talent show with Soldiers doing some dancing to their favorite music, or playing the guitar, and some karaoke. The show started with free popcorn for the

Soldiers and lots of laughter for those who needed to unwind from the hot day and relax with your fellow comrades. I had taken pictures of most of the show for next week's newsletter which would cover the July 4th Holiday in Iraq for HHC 601st ASB. The talent show ended with some good clean fun with everyone getting the chance to make others laugh. The next morning, July 3 2008, about 9:00AM, I was walking down to the laundry point to turn in my dirty uniforms, when a first sergeant stopped me by saying that he needed some help with a Soldier that had been found in his room. It's never good news when the mortuary affairs is asked to go to work, but he told me that this Soldier reported as a non-combat related incident, as I asked for the Soldiers name, his reply was that it was SPC Green, the Chaplains Assistant. My heart sank to my stomach with disbelief, and just couldn't believe that it was SPC Green. I called the Mortuary Affairs Collection Point on the COB (Contingency Operation Base), and told them that I would be over since I was representing the CAB. I arrived at the MACP, within thirty minutes the NCOIC and I drove over to the CSH (Combat Surgical Hospital), to escort the Soldiers remains to the MACP for further processing. Once the CID (Criminal Investigation Division), the agents took fingerprints and photos for the investigation. I looked at SPC Green, who always gave encouragement to other Soldiers in the HHC 601st ASB.

The investigation continues even after CID completed the fingerprints and photos. I left the mortuary affairs collection point and returned back to brief the Battalion Commander on the status of the deceased Soldier. I told the Commander that this is why I am here in this unit to take care of the deceased Soldiers. I could sense that he had confidence in handling the affairs for SPC Green. The weather was clear and there were no reports of any sandstorms coming so that the remains wouldn't be delayed for shipping. The flight arrangements were made through the MACP, which most of the time the U.S. Air Force's C-130 supports the missions to transport all U.S. Soldiers remains from most locations in Iraq to a U.S. Base in Kuwait. In the meantime, the crime scene was cleared for entry but the room had blood on the walls and ceiling. I told my 1SG, that my Soldier who is a mortuary affairs, and I would volunteer to remove the biohazard materials, sanitize the room, prior to inventorying SPC Green's personal effects. The next morning at 9:00AM, my Soldier and I walked into the room with red biohazard bags, mops, gloves, gowns and masks. We didn't want those who were close to SPC Green to help with the clean up, as some wanted but under these circumstances, the both of us have worked beside a Medical Examiner in Topeka, Kansas since 2004, and been on numerous crime scenes. It took us two days to clean the room, and additional five days to assist the officer during the personal effects inventory.

The mortuary affairs collection point NCOIC called the support operations office and left a message that SPC Green's remains will be shipping today at 1:30PM. I notified the Chaplains at Brigade, and the other Battalions of the departure time. We took a break from the inventory and went to the dining facility. We were sitting at the table eating when a Soldier approached to tell us that the C-130 was on its way and would be landing in twenty minutes. The airfield was on the other side of the COB, so we had no time to waste. There was the HHC 1SG, 2nd Lieutenant, SGT Dietzler, and I, having lunch. The four of us left the dining facility with a purpose, which took us ten minutes to get to the entrance of the airfield, only to see the MACP vehicle backing up to the rear of the Air Force C-130. The C-130's flight crew started preparing for the ramp ceremony, as we were walking across the airfield. The 1SG, Lieutenant, SGT Dietzler and I, stood in two equal ranks facing each other with some assistance from the flight crew to give us eight for a ramp ceremony. The U.S. Flag draped over the transfer case as the first Soldier slowly removes the case, as each Soldier in the formation grasps the transfer case. There were some passengers aboard that stood at attention to give the slow hand salute as SPC Green, was slowly making its way up the ramp of the C-130. The Soldiers rested the transfer case on the floor of the aircraft where it would remain until it reaches its destination. The Chaplains, and Chaplain Assistant's from each respective unit arrived about five minutes later, so since they had missed the ceremony, I didn't want to delay the evacuation of the remains, but the with the pilots permission, he allowed the Chaplains, and their Assistants to board the aircraft for a quick word of prayer. We boarded the C-130 from the crew's side door and to the rear of the plane, where the transfer case rested. The Chaplain's stood over this Soldier, with tears in their eyes and SPC Green's fellow comrades who knew of his encouraging words he shared with them and others during this deployment. I couldn't hold back the tears knowing that this was a Soldier, in the midst of this war he suffered from the same things that most Soldiers fight during these long and hard tours, the stress, depression, but I had one thing I had to do, which was to forgive him, and to leave the rest for God to decide.

There isn't much a Spouse, Child, or Soldier, can say when you send off your Son or Daughter off to war. When you get the letters from them telling you about life in Iraq, and that they miss home very much, and for mommy's to give their children a kiss goodnight from daddy, who is across the world fighting the war in Iraq or Afghanistan. The Soldiers who sleep two to three hours a night after coming off a patrol mission or guard duty, but from what I have experienced in my two tours in Iraq, it doesn't matter your job, or branch of service, I have seen those who have sacrificed everything, and those who wear the uniform every day, will never quit!

Chapter Four
"Operation PCS"

The 601st Combat Aviation Brigade returned from their fifteen month deployment on November 18th 2008. While the Soldiers were returning home to see their spouses, children, and extended families, I was looking to PCS (Permanent Change of Station), to Fort Lee, Virginia in March 2008. I did come home to a newly constructed home that my wife and I had bought while I was in Iraq. She moved into a thirty two hundred foot square home with four bedrooms, three full baths, which two were master bathrooms, and ours have a Jacuzzi. However, I would be trading that lifestyle with an apartment somewhere near Fort Lee, Virginia.

The most important thing besides moving from my home was the promotion of the books "BEYOND ENVY" and "THE HEART OF A SHEPHERD," on the following Saturday after Thanksgiving Day, at the Barnes & Noble Bookstore in Topeka, Kansas. I thought to myself, here I am surrounded by some of the greatest Authors in the world, and now I am promoting my books, which was the biggest thrill of my life. I even contacted a friend who led me to Deb Goodrich who worked for a local radio station, so I did the live interview a few days before appearing at the bookstore. The day of the signing I put on my tailored made Italian brown suit, and this couldn't have been possible without God, so I could share my story with others. As I entered the store had a table with the books all set up, the Barnes & Noble poster with my name and photo of myself. The customer relations manager at the B&N did a terrific job to make this an event that was a successful day at one of the largest book stores in the world.

I continued to promote the two books, just two weeks before Christmas at the Hastings Book Store in Manhattan, Kansas, where I lived so this would generate local attention and afterwards having the books available in the store on consignment.

In December we celebrated the Christmas Holiday season together and bringing in the New Year 2009.

About mid March, I started my PCS move to Fort Lee, Virginia, which would allow me to take thirty days of leave to spend a few weeks with my wife and children, before heading to the east coast.

I moved into a nine hundred foot square apartment, with two bedrooms, and rented for six hundred a month. I reported to Ft. Lee on April 10, 2009, where I was assigned to the 54th Quartermaster (Mortuary Affairs), unit for the next twenty four months, who deploys to Iraq for six month tours. After the first week in the unit, I was the Operations NCOIC, which was short lived for two weeks. In the month of May, I was reassigned as the military schools NCOIC, which lasted a week more than the first, which after I returned from celebrating Armed Forces Day, which is the last week of May, I had been selected as the 2nd Platoon Sergeant, which lasted to June 29, 2009. During the events as the Platoon Sergeant, I worked some long hours, leading, mentoring, training, and directing Soldiers. As a noncommissioned officer the thought of denying a leadership position isn't part of our backbone. We accept the challenge that molds us to becoming the best as we move to the next level of responsibility. I was a former Infantry Drill Sergeant, which goes back to the 1980's, as some called it "Old School," basic training, discipline, tougher physical fitness training, but times have changed as the new generations that are now among our military ranks have come with changes. No doubt everyday is a new monster, but that's what so great about being a noncommissioned officer, we have made a difference since 1775, like the great Sergeant Audie Murphy.

I had been the Platoon Sergeant for about thirty days, but little did I know that I still had some old wounds from my first Iraq deployment in 2006. I was experiencing sleep problems, stress, depression, and financial situations due to having to handle two households. There were months where I didn't even have money to buy food, or gas so I could get to work. I did get some assistance from military programs that had helped, but they just get you through till your next payday. Therefore, there were a lot of circumstances that were being piled on top of what I still holding deep inside of me, which eventually did come to the surface. The first incident occurred when I overslept and missed the Platoon Sergeant's meeting with the 1SG, which he or she puts out critical information that the Soldiers need to know. By the time I got to the Company's Physical Fitness formation, the 1SG gives the command "Fall In," this is followed by each Platoon Sergeant to have each squad leader give the report of all Soldiers in the squad, as their whereabouts. This information is what is given to the 1SG, for the daily status for the entire company. Well, as you can see, I wasn't at the meeting earlier and now showing up late to formation. After the formation the 1SG called me to the rear of the formation and he asked me what's going on with me. I told him that I am having trouble sleeping, and I thought I needed to see a doctor to correct this problem.

I made an appointment with Community Mental Health, but it wouldn't be until June 29, 2009.

A few weeks went by without any occurrences not until on an early Sunday morning, about 1:15AM, we had a mandatory formation for a unit that were deploying to Iraq for twelve months. I set my alarm to midnight so I would be ready, but again I was so exhausted that I didn't even hear the alarm. One of the squad leaders from my platoon called and asked where I was and that I missed the formation. At this time, I quickly became depressed, stressed so much that I was sweating, and anxiety.

The next day around noon, I was already emotional that I called my wife, and she told me to call the 1SG. I called the 1SG on his cell phone, by this time my emotions were noticeable to him, and then the red flags go up everywhere. The 1SG directed me to see Mental Health on Monday morning, which is exactly what I did the following day. Monday morning at 7:30, the clinic was opened for walk in appointments, so I checked in with the receptionist and waited for the Mental Health Specialist. I was sitting there for about twenty minutes, when the CMH Counselor asked me to come back to his office. As we sat in his office, he wanted to know how I was feeling today and what the reason is why I am here at CMH. My explanation was that I had been having some stress, depression, anxiety, as he could tell from the tone in my voice and the black circles under my eyes; I had some concerns that needed direct attention. I also mentioned that most of this was when I came home from Iraq in 2006. He then asked me that if going to a Hospital to get treatment. Without any hesitation, I volunteered myself to be admitted to a Hospital, knowing that I had not been the same person since returning home from the war.

Chapter Five

"Soldier, Take a Knee"

I was admitted to the Poplar Springs Behavioral Hospital in Petersburg, Virginia. This is more like a healthcare facility that provides a military wing for military Soldiers, who come from the surrounding states for treatment. The procedures were that you have to be escorted to the PSH, and once there you will be directed to a private room where you will wait for the admissions office to discuss the rules for visitations and complete the forms for billing to Tricare. I met the Admissions representative, who directed me to another office nearby, so she could finish the admission, and to get a patient Identification bracelet that had a small photo of me. The woman left the office to get some lunch for me from the cafeteria. When she returned to the office she escorted me to the military wing which every door has a security camera, and secured at all times. There I was introduced to the head nurse who then took me to a room with three beds where I would be sleeping. There I had to remove my ACU's (Army Combat Uniform), down to my underwear, so I did, which he removed my belt, boot laces, all sharp objects that could be used to harm myself. I thought that this was a little extreme, but its policy and it protects the other patients and staff. I could wear my Army PT uniform which I had with me but I asked how I would wear the shoes without the laces, he replied with zipped ties. I used a couple of zip ties to lace my shoes to keep them on my feet. The items were locked in a room, where I would have access to them when I needed to shave, with supervision. Here I was in the Hospital a Soldier with "Zipped Tied Boots," that had gone through horrific experiences during two tours in Iraq, and had written and published books. The other patients were sitting around the tables playing monopoly, cards, and some watching television. A few Soldiers introduced themselves to me almost immediately which made me feel more comfortable. I felt like this would take me a few days to get into the routine of my stay here at PSH. The schedule is filled with activities that are treatment related so this place didn't offer the horseback riding, shuffleboard, sitting out at pool side getting a tan. I was prescribed medication to help me sleep which is the one thing I was looking forward to doing since being here in Virginia. After a few days of PSH, I quickly become more aware of the routine of the heavy schedule and talking with the patients who where there for other reasons than PTSD. There were those who were alcoholics, those who were having problems with co dependency relationships, anger problems, but one thing we all had in common, was we were Soldiers. The military unit had seventeen patients when I first arrived, we participated in group therapy which is like an ethics class, where there is no right or wrong answer but we all shared our opinions which helped open the floor for the new patients that are reluctant to share their issues that brought them to PSH. I found that the group sessions were times for Soldiers to learn more about each owns issues and for some that allowed others to be later released from PSH. The atmosphere to those few patients seems like you're locked up, with no idea you're release date, a program that is there to help them, and so it's up to the individual to complete the treatment. In the first three days, I started writing some notes of what this experience in PSH meant to me and for those who have never received treatment for

PTSD. My stay in PSH, was just for eight days, but during that time I received the proper medical care, medications to stabilize me to where I can sleep and get me through the day, without feeling tired. We received three meals a day, and were given time to do physical fitness, and free time to call our families from the wing at no charge. The day of my release I couldn't wait to get home and get back to my previous routine, but without knowing that during my treatment at PSH, I learned something about myself and how I can cope with my PTSD, and now maybe help other Soldiers, since my treatment.

Chapter Six

"Road to Recovery"

The road to any recovery begins with a plan that gives the individual the proper tools and guidance to follow their plan, during a crisis. The plan is called a "Safety Plan"; it covers personal goals, special people in your life, physical and mental milestones. First, you don't have to be admitted to a Behavioral Hospital to use this safety plan and you don't need to pay a doctor office visit to get this prescribed. All you need is yourself, some 3x5 cards, pen, and a quiet place to think of your own personalized "Safety Plan." I will be discussing the safety plans outline in which it was intended to be utilized, like for example like baking a cake; first you make a list with the right ingredients to make the cake, so you make a shopping list. Then as you have acquired those ingredients you lay them out to ensure you haven't forgotten something. If you're brain is tired then you have everything. Now, we are ready to make our plan. Here are the steps you need to follow in order for you to get full use from your personalized safety plan.

Step One: Checks and Balances

What you were feeling at the time when you were going through the tough times. It could be your emotions, feeling guilty, depression, sad, responsibility, or anxiety.

Step Two: Outlets

There are three types of outlets for everyone; the first one is called "Physical Outlets", which are but not limited to, giving someone you love a hug, fishing with a relative or close friend, hitting the punching bag when you feel angered about something, writing a book, taking walks through the park. The second outlet is called "Mental Outlets, like reading your favorite book, playing a video game, spending time in prayer, putting puzzles together, keeping a journal of your daily thoughts. The third is called "Emotional Outlets," for instance having a good cry or laugh, intimacy with your spouse, visiting the children in the hospital, or the elderly in the nursing homes.

Step Three: Coping Skills

The things that you would do if you were feeling some anxiety, stressed which is those things you would do if you needed some time to yourself. Here are some examples, like talking with your spouse, calling an old friend, playing a round of golf, taking an afternoon nap, sitting in a Jacuzzi, listening to your favorite music artist.

Step Four: Someone to Talk With

These people have been there for you in a time of crisis. When you needed someone to come over when you needed a friend.

Step Five: PMCS

(Preventive Maintenance Checks and Services.)

These should be those people that are there to support you during your crisis. If your around those who are pulling you back to the old you, then you need to find an exit, and don't look back.

Step Six: Comforts

Here we have some ideas that will give you time to yourself, like having hot chicken soup on a cold day, watching old movies, breakfast in bed.

Step Seven: Spiritual

Visiting your local church, or talking with your priest of pastor, and donating to charity.

Step Eight: Aftercare

If you're taking medications, continue as doctor ordered. A change in your diet, exercise plan, massages therapy.

Step Nine: Call Rosters

Make a list of names of family or friends who you can call when you need them.

Step Ten: Touchstones

These personal items have special meaning to you. For example, your wedding pictures, newspaper articles about you or your children.

Step Eleven: Rewards

It's your day off from work, and you have nothing planned, so here are some ideas, having lunch with your spouse, or an evening dinner date, going to the movies, buying yourself a new outfit.

Final Step: Feedback

Set goals for yourself; schedule your time using a daily planner, listen to those who love you, that can tell you that you've made some great progress, and those who can give you an honest opinion, even if it hurts, as long as they do it out of love.

In Conclusion:

This book has given me the chance to express the actual events that I have experienced and since wanted to share them with others who may be dealing with PTSD. I encourage you to find the resources available to you before it's too late. My writing comes from the heart as is in all my books that I have written, which are still published today. I wish all those who read this book or others, God Bless!